POST MARKETING

PHARMACOEPIDEMIOLOGY

Dr. Ravi Humbarwadi

Quality Lead in a Global Corporate

CONTENT

1. INTRODUCTION

2. NON-INTERVENTIONAL STUDIES

3. PASS

4. POST MARKETING PHARMACOEPIDEMIOLOGY – THE OBJECTIVES

5. MONITORING POST-MARKETING SAFETY

6. EVALUATION OF SAFETY SIGNALS

7. RISK MANAGEMENT

8. COMPARATIVE EFFECTIVENESS AND SAFETY

9. ENCePP

10. GUIDELINES FOR EPIDEMIOLOGY STUDIES

INTRODUCTION

Definition

Pharmacoepidemiology is the scientific study of the utilization and effect (effectiveness and safety) of drugs involving large number of people by using epidemiological methods.

Epidemiologic studies are conducted to predict probability of outcomes of parameters such as:

a. Therapeutic efficacy
b. Occurrence of adverse effects
c. Dose - Duration- Response curve
d. Impact of genetic modifications on drug efficacy and safety
e. Effects of non-compliance and assessment of programs aimed at enhancing compliance in selected population.
f. Drug-drug interaction outcomes

1. Analytic:

    A. Observational studies - Case-control and cohort studies.

    B. Experimental studies - Clinical trials.

In analytical studies hypotheses are tested by evaluation of the drug with a comparator drug. Comparison with a standard drug allows the sponsor to assess the advantages and the disadvantages of their drug. It gives a perspective of the benefits versus risk of their drug with regards to current accepted therapy.

2. Descriptive: Disease incidence and prevalence, and drug exposure are studied in defined populations. The study of disease incidence, prevalence and drug usage allows the sponsor to evaluate the parameters under which the drug is used and the factors that might be affecting the effectiveness and safety of the drug.

NON – INTERVENTIONAL STUDIES

According to the EU article 2c, non-interventional studies are defined as "Studies where the medicinal products are prescribed in the usual manner in accordance with the terms of the marketing authorization. The assignment of the patient to a particular therapeutic strategy is not decided in advance by a trial protocol but falls within current practice and the prescription of the medicine is clearly separated from the decision to include the patient in the study."

Non-interventional studies:

- Epidemiologically analyzed.
- The drugs given to the subject are as per medical prescription.
- There is no protocol for giving the treatment.
- The laboratory tests are as per medical requirement by the clinician.
- Approved drugs and medical devices are used.

.

Non-interventional studies include database analysis which is retrospective in nature (secondary use of data) – claims, electronic medical records and hospital databases. Non-interventional studies which are prospective in nature (primary data collection) are the prospective observational studies and registries.

The common study designs used in the non-interventional studies are case-control, cross-sectional and cohort.

The three common study designs used in non-interventional studies are:

- Cohort-studies
- Case-control studies
- Cross-sectional studies

Cohort study

In cohort studies, a group of people within a population is observed over a period of time to identify who experiences the same significant event or treatment. This type of design is most useful to identify incidence, cause and prognosis. They measure events in chronological order and hence they can be used to identify cause and effect.

Cohort studies can be done prospectively, retrospectively, or using cross-sectional methods. Comparison studies between two groups is also possible – one group with drug under observation compared to a control group without the drug.

Cross-sectional study

Cross-sectional study designs are used when studying one or more variables within a given population at one point in time. Such studies are useful for establishing associations rather than causality and for determining prevalence, rather than incidence.

Case control study

Case control studies are used to compare a group with a certain medical condition with a control group. Case control studies are often retrospective studies. The control group is generally from the same population and has similar age and gender characteristics but has not developed the medical condition under observation. Case control studies attempt to identify potential outcome predictors.

They are used to generate hypotheses that can be further tested using the prospective cohort or other appropriate study designs.

Family-based case-control type design uses related persons as the control group and is useful to analyze both early as well as late onset medical conditions. The analysis is done using conditional logistic regression. Group with parents is preferred for study of birth defects or early onset medical conditions.

- Preferred for analysis of
  Rare medical conditions
  Conditions with long duration between exposure and outcome

- When compared to cross-sectional studies lesser subjects are required to carry out the case control studies

Medical records are required to confirm the exposure. In the absence of medical documents the study has to rely on the memory of the subjects with regards to exposure. This design may have bias such as selection and recall bias.

PASS

A post-authorisation study becomes a post authorization safety study (PASS) when it has the following objectives:

- Quantification of risk

Incidence rate of the adverse event under study in comparison to a population without exposure.

Incidence rate of the adverse event with the study drug in comparison to a population that is being treated with a comparator drug.

Evaluation of co- factors that could have led to increase in the occurrence of adverse event.

Evaluation of factors that could impact and change the drug effect.

- Assessment of risk associated with long-term drug usage.

Assessment of risk associated with the drug use in special patient populations such as pregnant women, pediatric, geriatric and liver or kidney dysfunctional patient populations.

The participation of these populations in the clinical trial might have been minimal. So data obtained during clinical trials is usually insufficient to quantify the safety of drug usage in such populations.

- Confirmation of the absence of risks.

- Conducts research on factors that impact drug safety including study of the indication, dosage, co-morbidities and concomitant medications, inadvertent or intentional medication errors and off–label uses. Such research comes under the category of drug utilization studies.

- Conducts follow up study to find out whether risk minimization measures have been useful and are delivering the results as per expectations.

Register in EUPAS.

To make the conduct and results of a PASS study available for wider scrutiny the details of a non-interventional PASS should be posted in the EU electronic register of post-authorization studies (EU PAS Register).

The study should have a protocol based on scientific principles developed by professionals with the required scientific qualification, background and expertise. The protocol should be registered in EU PAS registry prior to initiation of the study. Amendments, ongoing reports and the final report should be updated generally within two weeks after their finalization.

Reporting Adverse Events

It is the responsibility of the MAH to monitor the study data. Adverse events that are detected should be reported to the regulatory authorities within the regulatory timelines.

Risk - Benefit

A thorough risk-benefit analysis should be conducted by the MAH. Data suggesting new risks associated the drug use is classified as an 'Emerging Safety Issue' and should be reported to the regulatory authorities.

Final Report

The final study report should be submitted generally within a year of the end date of the data collection.

Publication

A publication policy should be prepared prior to start of the study to enable efficient publication of the study result.

POST MARKETING PHARMACOEPIDEMIOLOGY

The Objectives

Monitor Post-marketing Safety

Identify Safety Signals

Risk management plan (RMP) and Re-check the RMP

Effectiveness and Safety Studies with Comparator

MONITORING POST-MARKETING SAFETY

A. To identify new adverse events that were missed or were not revealed during phase 1-3 of the clinical trials.

B. Study of safety issues in special populations.

C. To gain more clarity of known adverse effects:

- Changes in the severity or frequency of the known adverse events
- Dose-response and duration – response relationship
- Drug-drug or drug - disease interactions
- Medication errors and off- label use
- Effect of chronic and long term drug use

The phase 1-3 of clinical trials are conducted is in a few thousands of subjects. But post approval the drug is prescribed and dispensed to the general population which is many times larger. During comparison studies in phase 3 many times placebo is used as a comparator while it seems to be a better idea to compare toxicity of new drugs to standard drugs rather than with a comparator. In actual clinical practice drugs may be used in doses, frequencies and in patient groups not studied in the trials. Further, the patients may be taking many other concomitant medications and may be having complicated medical history predisposing to newer drug-drug and drug-disease interactions that can have unpredictable outcomes. Physicians may be prescribing for off - label uses.

On the other hand there may be medication errors such as overdose (accidental or intentional), inappropriate regimens, skipped doses, and drug abuse.

1. Spontaneous Reports

Spontaneous adverse drug reaction reports can be obtained from:

- Pharmacovigilance databases
  -FAERS,
  -Eudravigilance
  -WHO Vigibase (WHO global database).
  VigiBase is the WHO global ICSR database. VigiBase contains Individual Safety Case Reports submitted from member countries in the WHO Programme for International Drug Monitoring since 1968.
- Poison control centers provide accidental or intentional drug poisoning and drug intoxication cases.
- Vaccine surveillance
- Teratology information centers
- Literature

2. Sentinel surveillance

It is a reporting system based on selected institutions or individual that provide regular, complete reports on one or more diseases occurring.

It may be the best type of surveillance if more intensive investigation of each case is necessary to collect the necessary data.

3. Post-approval safety studies

PASS - A post authorization study carried out specifically to evaluate the safety aspect or assess the results of risk minimization activities with regards to an approved drug.

A PASS may be conducted voluntarily or may be conducted to fulfill a mandatory requirement ordered by a regulatory authority.

A post-authorization safety study (PASS) can be mandated in the European Union during the initial marketing authorization application or during the post-authorization phase by the EMEA or the national regulatory authorities, if in their judgment there are risks that require further monitoring. This mandatory requirement is an outcome of an extensive benefit- risk analysis and should include the objectives to be met and the timeline for completion of the study. The regulatory authority may give suggestions regarding the population and design of the study, and the safety issues that need to be addressed.

All mandatory post-authorization safety studies need to be incorporated in the RMP (risk management plan) and their results should be mentioned in the periodic safety reports that are submitted to the regulatory authorities by the sponsor.

4. Registries

A system that uses observational study methods to collect data of a population that is specified by a disease or usage of a particular drug. Hence, we can have either product or disease registries.

Advantages Of Registry

Large patient numbers that are enrolled in a registry can help uncover rare adverse events.

Study subjects are heterogeneous and this allows a study of drug use in a variety of patients.

Effect of different concomitant medications and co-morbidities can be observed.

Registries - Example

Pregnancy Registry

A pregnancy exposure registry is an observational study that actively collates data on drug exposure during pregnancy and effect if any on pregnancy outcomes.

Pregnancy exposure registries differ from other post-marketing surveillance techniques, such as birth defect registries and spontaneous reporting, in that the pregnancy registry is a prospective study. The pregnant women are registered prior to pregnancy outcome.

If it is likely that the drug will be used during pregnancy as therapy for a new or chronic disease such as hypertension, gestational diabetes and epilepsy that occur during pregnancy then a pregnancy registry study will be extremely useful to the sponsor and the sponsor should initiate such a study.

Pregnancy is often an exclusion criterion for clinical trials. If a subject becomes pregnant during the trial, study drug therapy is discontinued and the subject is withdrawn from the study. Therefore pregnancy registries play a significant role in the assessment which is not possible to do in clinical trials. If not evidence of risk of the drug they are useful in providing evidence of lack of risk or margin of safety during pregnancy. The registry is useful in detection of early safety signals and to study factors that could affect the risk such as dose, drug regimen, route of administration and maternal factors.

> Pregnancy Registry To Be Started.
>
> At the time of start of marketing of a new drug.
>
> At the time when a new indication is approved.
>
> FDA usually asks for a mandatory registry study during the post marketing phase.
>
> FDA may seek a registry study for a drug at pre- approval stage.
>
> When trends obtained from spontaneous reporting indicate potential pregnancy – related risks.

The design of a registry should be aligned to its objectives which can be open-ended or could be testing pre-specified hypotheses.

A general multidrug registry, such as a teratogen information service, collects information on different drugs used in different indications during pregnancy. Multidrug registries may be more economical and collect information of several drugs in the same time as compared to registries.

Pregnancy registries are preferred as initial study. Other studies such as case control studies and studies using automated databases may be done to confirm any safety signals that arise from a registry.

Case control studies can:

A. Evaluate rare adverse birth events
B. Be used when long-term follow- up is required
C. Establish the degree of causality between the drug and the risk.

Case control studies can be designed in such a manner that they can be a sub - part of a pregnancy registry.

Studies using automated databases can provide information on range of issues including maternal exposure and maternal and infant outcomes. Automated studies are feasible when the drug is accepted and used by a large pool of population so that enough reports show up in the automated databases.

Reporting of Registry Events.

The FDA considers pregnancy registry reports as actively solicited data. So, serious adverse events (SAE) which are unexpected with a reasonable possibility that the drug was the cause of the adverse event (causality) have to be submitted within the regulatory timeline of 15 days by the marketing authorization holder (MAH).

Pregnancy exposure registries that are not conducted by the marketing authorization holder do not have to mandatorily submit adverse event reports.

The sponsor of a registry which is either a pre or post marketing requirement by the FDA should submit an annual status report.

1. Pregnancy Registry

Example A: Pregnancy Registry of Drugs used in Gestational Diabetes.

This type of pregnancy registry monitors exposure to brand name-specific drugs used in gestational diabetes. Reporting of exposed pregnancies is voluntary and is initiated by the pregnant woman or her health care provider (HCP). Once registered the follow ups are done via the health care providers. The obstetric HCP informs regarding maternal risk factors and outcome of the pregnancy. The pediatric HCP informs about birth defects and developmental milestones at pre-specified intervals.

Merck Pregnancy Registry Program of Janumet (sitagliptin phosphate plus metformin hydrochloride) in the treatment of Type 2 Diabetes.

The Pregnancy Registry for Janumet receives voluntary reports from HCPs or from pregnant women who have been treated with Janumet during pregnancy. The women are enrolled in the registry and their pregnancies are followed with the HCP.

Example B: Humira (Adalimumab) Pregnancy Exposure Registry: OTIS Rheumatoid Arthritis in Pregnancy Project.

The study type was observational. The study design was an observational model – cohort and the time perspective was prospective.

The aim of the study was to evaluate the possible teratogenic effect of these medications which are used in the treatment of autoimmune diseases such as Crohn's disease and rheumatoid arthritis during pregnancy and to follow live born infants for one year after birth.

Primary Outcome Measure: Major malformations throughout pregnancy and upto 1 year in the baby.

Secondary Outcome Measures include:

- Minor malformations that are detected at the time of dysmorphological examination.

- Pregnancy outcomes such as spontaneous abortion, stillbirth, and preterm delivery for which monitoring is done throughout pregnancy

- Fetal and Infant follow-ups done throughout pregnancy and upto 1 year monitor pre- and post-natal fetal and infant growth and development.

Among the cohorts in the study were the exposure and the matched disease comparison cohort.

Exposure cohort
Pregnant women with a current diagnosis of rheumatoid arthritis including juvenile or Crohn's disease who have used adalimumab in the first trimester of pregnancy for any length of time from the date of conception.

Matched Diseased Comparison Cohort
Pregnant women with a current diagnosis of rheumatoid arthritis including juvenile or Crohn's disease who have not used adalimumab or any tumour necrosis factor (TNF) antagonist in pregnancy.

2. Medical Condition / Disease Registry

Example A: A Renal Allograft Study

The renal allograft registry maintained records of patients post renal allograft. It was useful in establishing that recurrent disease was a significant problem after renal transplantation and was associated with less than optimal graft survival.

Example B: The Carotid Artery Stenting with Emboli Protection Surveillance Post-Marketing Study (CASES-PMS)

This study was initiated to evaluate the outcomes of carotid artery stent procedures for the treatment of obstructive artery disease in the periapproval setting, including the use of a detailed training program for physicians not experienced in carotid artery stenting.

The registry was a multicenter, prospective, observational study designed to assess stenting outcomes in relation to the outcomes of the SAPPHIRE trial (historic comparison group). The study enrolled 1,493 patients from 74 sites, using inclusion and exclusion criteria that matched those of the historic comparison group.

The analysis revealed that the training program in carotid stenting equipped clinicians with requisite skills and allowed them to attain results that matched the results of the experts during the clinical trials.

The registry could provide data to analyze the safety of the device and also the effectiveness of training specialist clinicians.

As you can see such registries are powerful mechanisms to arrive at important scientific conclusions that have an impact on how a drug should be used, the risk factors and any mitigation measures that need to be taken or awareness programs that need to be initiated to improve drug safety and effectiveness.

5. Automated Databases

The automated databases provide an extensive population, a variety of drugs and drug classes and are less expensive.

Claims database

The claims database refers to the claims documentation provided by clinics, hospitals and doctors to insurance companies.

- Incidence of strokes in patients using a particular drug.

Claims database is the preferred choice for this type of data. The hospital database may have more details such as surgical procedures done (with explanation of the procedure), treatment given on a day to day basis, details of all the lab investigations carried out etc. Here, the objective is to just find the incidence vis-a vis usage of a particular drug and claims database can provide an extensive database and a varied choice of population. The data is for billing purpose and it may be incomplete with regards to in-depth medical or surgical details.

Electronic medical records database

The electronic medical record (EMR) of the patient includes co-morbidities, concomitant and past drugs clinical examination, diagnosis, medical therapy and surgical procedures alongwith laboratory results.

- Prevalence of syncope in chronic hypertensive patients managed in the primary care setting.

The EMR has more outpatient details. Such medical conditions that are treated as outpatient settings are typically available in the EMR of the patient.

Hospital database

The hospital databases are the repository of the reports and medical condition of patients when they undergo hospitalization due to any medical or surgical reason.

- Hospital length of stay when a particular drug was used in comparison with another drug.

To obtain accurate information of hospitalization the hospital database would be the preferred option.

In order to implement an end to end epidemiological study more often than not several of the above mentioned studies have to be used.

6. Drug Utilization Studies

Drug utilization studies are conducted to identify the extent and nature of drug exposure in large populations. These studies reveal the prescription patterns and drug usage as they happen in actual clinical practice. The special populations that are not part of the clinical trials can also be part of drug utilization studies.

Pattern Of Drug Use In A Population:

- The extent of drug exposure: how many patients and how much of drug is used.

- Drug profile : Drug under study, comparator, other drugs in same class – type, formulation, route

- Trends : Demographic, geographic, shifts in prescription patterns

- Costs

Quality Of Drug Use

Drug audit is done and the practice of drug use is evaluated against the standard guidelines for
- Drug prescribed: Whether the drug which is prescribed is as per the accepted recommendations or is there difference. Is the difference due to lack of knowledge of current practice. If so would focused training bridge the gap between actual practice and the standard guidelines?

- Drug cost: If costly drugs are prescribed is there a medical reason for this. Could the medical condition have been treated with a less costly drug. At what lowest cost could the medical condition be treated with no compromise on treatment outcome?

- Drug dosage - factors for variations in dosage.

- Drug – drug interactions: Did the doctor consider potential drug-drug interactions when prescribing. Was the doctor aware of drug- drug interactions? Awareness in the population with regards to benefits, risks and costs when a particular drug is used.

Decision Factors

What factors decide the choice of drug to be used in a particular condition?

- Demographic factors

- Doctor factors: Qualification, experience and any other factors that impact the prescription.

- Drug: Benefits, risks and cost.

Final Outcome

Benefit to the patient's health, any risk posed by the drug and the cost implications of therapy to the patient.

DRUG UTILISATION STUDIES

Can be used to examine the relationship between recommended treatment guidelines and actual clinical practice.

Over as well as under use of drugs can be detected

Can help to detect drug abuse by noting whether patients are taking escalating dose regimens or there is inappropriate repeat prescribing.

Can be used to monitor the effect of regulatory changes and media focus on drug usage.

Can be used to develop estimates of the cost of drugs. The evaluation of the economic impact of clinical care and medical technology has evolved into the study of how pharmacotherapeutics affects healthcare resource utilization (pharmacoeconomics). Drug utilization research provides insight into the efficiency of drug use - whether a certain therapy provides value for money. This is used in optimizing health care budgets.

Denominator can be estimated. This allows calculation of rates of outcomes.

Drug utilization studies have various sources of information ranging from wholesale information to prescription registers in clinics. Drug utilization studies can be database studies or may employ primary data collection methodology.

Drug Utilization Research

Identify early signals of irrational use of drugs. Analysis and recommend steps to be taken to discontinue such irrational practices.

Drug utilization practices between different geographical, local or ethnic regions or at different times within the same population should be studied. Regional differences in drug use and trends that may inadvertently develop over a period of time may have both a medical and cost impact. The differences should be identified and corrective actions should be implemented so that the benefits of recommended guidelines are available across populations and at all times. Standardization of medical practice with regards to drug prescription should be established.

Identify undesirable patterns of drug use and use of undesirable drugs (lack of awareness of guidelines, intentional usage of undesirable drugs due to commercial considerations, compromise on cost due to lack of purchasing power by the patient) .

Ex: Opioid prescribing in emergency departments (ED): the prevalence of potentially inappropriate prescribing and misuse

Prevalence of potential opioid misuse and inappropriate prescription practices in a large and insured population in the emergency department. (Logan et al, 2013).

Study regarding the impact of regulatory changes or modification in insurance reimbursement process.

Ex: Utilization patterns of Antihyperuricemic Agents Following Safety Announcement on Allopurinol and Benzbromarone by Taiwan Food and Drug Administration

The outpatient prescriptions of 4 antihyperuricemic agents were extracted from a longitudinal cohort dataset with 1 000 000 individuals randomly sampled from the National Health Insurance Research Database in Taiwan. Utilization patterns of antihyperuricemic agents before and after the regulatory policy modification (safety information and labeling changes) in the year 2005 was studied. (Chen et al, 2014).

Study of the beneficial and deleterious effects of promotional campaigns

Study of the educational, social and economic status of a population and the drug use pattern.

Follow-up studies

Prescribers may change to other drugs that may also be undesirable. The total cost to society may remain the same or may even increase if more expensive or undesirable drugs are prescribed. So follow up studies are needed to ensure that prescribes follow standard recommendations.

Drug Use Patterns – Prevent Withdrawal of the Drug from the Market.

- Trends of use over a period of time. Factors that influence this trend. Once the mechanism of change in drug use is understood plans can be implemented to restart the correct trend.
- Comparison of drug usage habits with standard guidelines. If there is a gap this can be provided to the doctor as an awareness program so that corrective action can be initiated.
- Percentage of occurrence of adverse event – number of reports divided by the population exposed with regards to age group, specified indications and specified dosages.
- In some case just increasing the awareness on the labeled indications, contraindications and recommended dosage regimens may lead to correct drug use pattern.

Medicaid Drug Utilization Review (DUR) Program

The Medicaid Drug Utilization Review (DUR) Program strives for safety through state managed drug utilization systems that coordinate with the Medicaid Management Information Systems (MMIS). Medicaid DUR is a two-phase process. In the first phase the electronic monitoring system data mines the prescription drug claims for therapeutic duplication, drug-disease contraindications, incorrect dosage or duration of treatment, drug allergy, misuse and abuse

For the Medicaid program fraud, misuse and abuse are focus areas. Fraud hotlines, pain management and corrective case management programs have been initiated as measures to tackle some of the problems.

EVALUATION OF SAFETY SIGNALS

Stages of Signal Detection

Signal Generation: Identifies all suspected and unexpected adverse events. Thousands of adverse events or event pairs are collected. This is obtained after data mining of databases such as FAERS, VAERS, Eudravigilance and WHOVigibase.

Signal Refinement: Evaluation identifies adverse event pairs of interest. Active surveillance analysis of coded automated databases are useful in refining signals.

Signal Evaluation: In depth evaluation of a single pair. Co–factors leading to the adverse events and in-depth assessment of individual case is done to accept or refute the signal.

1. **Spontaneous Reports**

Adverse event reports, medication errors and product quality complaints are obtained through spontaneous reporting by both healthcare professionals – doctors, pharmacists and nurses and consumers – patients or patient's relatives.

The advantage of spontaneous reporting is that it allows comparison of events occurring after intake of the sponsor's drug with other standard drug (comparator).

Spontaneous reporting of adverse events is the most common methodology to generate signals of new or rare adverse events. It is useful in hypothesis generation that may require further analysis.

The disadvantages are:

Under or Over reporting – Since spontaneous reports may be reported by consumers who may not have scientific background it may result in under reporting i.e; not reporting events because they may be non-serious or not reporting serious events because they may have resolved. On the other hand over reporting may happen for instance if medical history is reported as an event.

Lack of Information – Lack of medical details which are required to conduct a proper analysis since the spontaneous reports from consumers are not always received in the CIOMS format or through Medwatch. Even if they are received through such formats these formats may be incomplete.

The total number of subjects actually consuming the drug under study which would have enabled the calculation of the percentage of occurrence of the event in the given population is not possible to be estimated.

2. Sentinel Surveillance

Sentinel surveillance is an active surveillance system for monitoring drug safety. It can refine signals and determine whether there is evidence of association. Sentinel surveillance can help decide whether a signal is true or false and produced by bias, confounding, or error.

3. Automated Databases

Longitudinal claims databases, electronic medical records or hospital databases.

RISK MANAGEMENT

Risk Management

:

(Risk Specification)

Evaluation of a product's risk and specify the risk - benefit

(Risk Minimization Plan)

Plan to minimize the risks without affecting the benefit

(RMP Assessment and Modification)

Monitor and modify the RMP as required to improve the risk-benefit balance.

The role of epidemiology in risk management:

Risk specification

The risk can be specified by comparing the rates of adverse events of the drug with the baseline incidence rates of adverse events in a population.

Sources of data for finding the baseline events and events after initiation of the drug are:

- Published literature
- Pooled clinical trial data
- Trial extensions
- Electronic health databases (insurance claims data or electronic medical records)
- Observational studies (prospective, retrospective cohort studies)

RMP

- The RMP can be implemented and modified based on the analysis from the following types of studies
- Spontaneous reports
- Signal management
- Clinical studies: These can be established to gather more information of specific risks
- Observational studies
- Post-authorization safety studies

COMPARATIVE EFFECTIVENESS AND SAFETY

Comparing effectiveness and risk of drug therapy used for the prevention, diagnosis or treatment during actual clinical practice. Such an evaluation can help to quantify a drug's performance with regards to efficacy and safety with comparator drugs which are already accepted and used.

Comparative effectiveness research (CER) in the USA is coordinated by The Patient Centered Outcomes Research Institute (PCORI). There is enormous expectation from the sponsors to provide comparative data. The sources for such data are the post marketing studies, prospective observational (registries) and retrospective observational research (databases).

CER helps the patients as well as the prescribers to take informed decisions with regards to drug therapy. Epidemiology is at the forefront in the evolution from purely reporting adverse events to addressing patient needs and value derived from a specific drug therapy when compared to other options.

Example of a CER study using automated databases and literature.

1. Automated Databases: Searches are conducted with regards to the drugs. The drugs names may be coded/hidden during the conduct of the comparative study.

2. Literature: Data for the drug under study and the comparator is obtained after a literature search.

Ex: The adverse effect profile and efficacy of divalproex sodium compared with valproic acid: a pharmacoepidemiology study. (Zarate CA Jr et al.1999).

Information of 150 patients who had been treated with divalproex sodium was gathered from the medical records and compared with the same number treated with valproic acid. The drug names were hidden for the purpose of the study. Pre-specified demographic and clinical data points were compared.

ENCePP

The European Network of Centres for Pharmacoepidemiology and Pharmacovigilance (ENCePP)

ENCePP is a network of more than 170 research centers and healthcare data providers with an objective of enhancing the effectiveness of post-authorization drug monitoring. ENCePP encourages the conduct of multicentre and independent safety and risk versus benefit studies.

The ENCePP Study Seal

ENCePP aims to promote high standards of conducting studies through the 'ENCePP Study Seal'. This seal is only awarded to sponsors who meet its well defined study criteria.

- The study should be done for the purpose of scientific research or public health.
- The focus of the study should not be to churn out data to increase drug sales.
- The study design should not be pre-conceived to achieve pre-specified results.
- The study protocol should be clear, straight forward and should recommend scientifically based methodologies that are aligned to meet the stated objectives.

- The sponsor and the investigator contracts or agreements should have utmost clarity on all issues and should lay down the responsibility of the investigator, remuneration, methodology of analysis and publication policy.
- Remuneration should be as per the protocol and for conducting the study and not for achieving a specified study result
- The study is registered in the ENCePP E-Register of Studies (EU PAS Register) prior to its start. This makes all information regarding the study available to the public.
- The study results are published in the ENCePP E-Register of Studies (EU PAS Register) within the specified timelines.

GOOD PHARMACOEPIDEMIOLOGY PRACTICES

The ISPE Guidelines for Good Pharmacoepidemiology Practices (GPP) lay down the best practices for the planning, conduct, and evaluation of pharmacoepidemiologic research. The GPP was initiated in 1996. In 2004 it was revised and included risk management, guidelines on regulatory reporting of individual cases and aggregate data and pharmacoeconomic activities. The second revision was in April 2007.

The GPP guidelines include:

- Protocol
- Responsibilities, Personnel, Facilities, Resource Commitment
- Conduct of the study
- Communication
- Reporting of Adverse Events
- Archiving

Pharmacoepidemiology studies should follow established guidelines to ensure that the study is conducted on a scientific basis and the results are authentic, accurate and unbiased.

The Protocol

The study should have a protocol based on scientific principles developed by professionals with the requisite qualification and expertise. The protocol can be modified during the conduct of the study.

Protocol Title and version

Names, qualification, affiliations, contact details of the principal investigator and co-investigators.　Name and contact details of the sponsor.

Introduction

Introduction and abstract of the protocol. Significant milestones with expected duration of meeting these milestones.

Study objective and measure of outcomes

Primary and secondary outcomes and measures of the outcome s should be described. The scientific basis of the research and its objectives. Hypotheses and whether the hypotheses are based on preliminary study.

Review of Literature

Literature review of pre-clinical, clinical trials and epidemiological research along with the conclusions of earlier research.

Study Design

Research design chosen. Provide the rationale for using the particular design over other designs. Inclusion exclusion criteria should be listed and the population should be defined. If comparator population is involved it should be defined. Duration of the study and duration of specific workflow processes to be detailed.

Data management.

The entire process of data management should be explained. Testing of data collection methods, training of data collection and data management staff, the hard ware, data analysis and statistical programs that will be used should be detailed. Metrics, categorizations, output format of results. Process for identification of missing and erroneous data.

Security of the data should be ensured. Access should be limited to authorized individuals. Document encryption should be undertaken. Data back up should be built in.

Process of ensuring accuracy and quality of data.

Process of authentication of data.

Process of validation of the outcomes.

Certification of clinical and laboratory facilities.

Statistical Analysis Plan.

The statistical procedures required to calculate point estimates, confidence intervals, risk ratios and any specified parameters.

The study size and statistical precision.

Ethics

Issue of confidentiality, treatment of adverse events, and study termination.

Publication

Communicating of the results is a very important function of the sponsor.

Quantitative measures in the results section using point estimates and confidence intervals preferably graphically. Results of safety studies should include both the relative and absolute risk estimates.

The individuals responsible for publication to be specified and are more often than not the principal investigator or the sponsor.

Amendments to the protocol.

Amendments should be documented with the reason and date of amendment.

Roles

The roles and responsibilities for conduct of the study should be described. When a study is outsourced timelines for completion of the study, data access rights, monitoring and publication responsibilities should be specified and documented in a signed legally binding agreement.

Personnel

All staff should possess the requisite qualification and experience and should be provided the necessary training required for their roles.

.

Study Conduct

The principal investigator is responsible for the study conduct.

The reason for premature study termination should be done only if there is a valid medical, scientific or ethical reason. This should be documented.

The sponsor and investigator should discuss all aspects which would warrant study termination even prior to start of the study and this should be well documented.

Protection of Human Subjects

Approval of the study by an Institutional Review Board (IRB) or Independent Ethics Committee (IEC) is required for studies with humans.

Informed consent by the subject is required when there is a risk to the subject or which have patient identifiers. With regards to patient identifiers measures to maintain confidentiality should be taken.

Study Reports

Document the requirement for an interim report. Interim reports and timing of the interim reports such reports can be initially discussed in the protocol itself.

The final report is done at the end of the study. It discusses the aims of the study – open ended or pre - specified hypothesis that is being tested, study design, results, limitations and its effects on results and the conclusion.

The final interpretation based on the statistical and medical evaluation of data; tables, graphs, and illustrations are required to give a visual display and also makes it easy to grasp the context.

Comment on the implication of the results.

The commonly reported statistical measures are risks, rates, risk or rate differences, and risk or rate ratios. It is preferred to state both the unadjusted and adjusted results. Estimation is preferred to tests of statistical significance.

Adverse Event Reporting

Individual case reporting: In prospective cohort (registry) and other prospective studies the adverse events that occur should be reported as individual case reports in an expedited manner within the regulatory timelines.

In the case-control and other retrospective studies which involve analysis of a series cases the findings are reported in the study reports and form part of aggregate reporting.

Archive

Archival of data should enable both storage and retrieval. An index sould be prepared that has a list of the archived content and location as well as the content that are not archived. Access should be given only to authorized staff and should be monitored.

The archive should be maintained for at least five years after final report or first publication of study results (whichever is later).

The archive should contain:

Signed institutional review board documents

The protocol

Final report

All source data

Master computer data file

Standard operating procedures

Location of all computer programs and statistical procedures

Signed informed consent forms

Quality assurance certifications

Documentation of the study result communication

STROBE

The Strengthening the Reporting of Observational Studies in Epidemiology (STROBE) program provides guidelines on the information that needs to be included in an observational study.

THE PHARMACOEPIDEMIOLOGY INTERVIEW

www.gipv.net

CERTIFICATE COURSE IN PHARMACOEPIDEMIOLOGY

www.gipv.net

INDUSTRY RELEVANT CERTIFICATION

www.gipv.net

DO YOU WANT TO TRY

THE PHARMACOEPIDEMIOLOGY
INTERVIEW.

www.gipv.net

Get that Better Job. Make a Career.

Helps you in Job Interviews.